Intermittent Fasting:

A Quick and Easy Guide for Beginners: The Secrets of Fat Burning, Rapid Weight Loss, and a Healthy Lifestyle.

Table of Contents

About Sarah Maddington

Sarah Maddington was born and raised in Manchester, UK. She is a Weight-Loss coach, Dietitian, Professional Chef and a mother of two. After finishing high school, she moved to London to pursue her dreams to study culinary.

In the past, Sarah was very overweight and suffered many health problems. She struggled with weight issues and found it difficult to maintain the balance between her career and her health.

It wasn't until after giving birth to her eldest daughter Sally, did she realise that she had to take her health more seriously if she wanted to become a role model for her children.

She lost 57 pounds in 6 months. Today, she wants to inspire beautiful people around the world to take control of the health so they can get back the life they deserve.

Introduction

You may be wondering what intermittent fasting is. Many people believe that it means that they can't eat for days on end, dealing with hunger pangs, but this just isn't the case. It's just a diet regime where you eat and fast within the day itself. It doesn't tell you what type of food you can consume, but just when you're able to actually eat. There are a few different intermittent fasting approaches out there. The body naturally fasts while we sleep, but with intermittent fasting you're prolonging this fast even after you wake up. Usually people start by eliminating breakfast from their daily routine, which would mean your first meal is usually eaten around midday. The second meal would be later in the evening.

One of the most popular intermittent fasting method is where you extend it to a 16/18 method, where you minimize your eating to eight hours. The fasting period you end up with is sixteen hours, but there are different types of intermittent fasting out there, which we'll cover in this book. You'll even learn about water fasting and other liquid fasting methods. Intermittent fasting isn't for everyone, but this book will take you through how to use intermittent fasting safely to reach your goals and pick the method that works best for you. You'll even learn how to adjust your intermittent fasting method so that you feel healthy and happy in the long term.

How it Works

It's important to understand how your body processes food if you want to understand how intermittent fasting actually work. When following the USDA's food pyramid, then body enters into a fed state. This means that your body has a high level of nutrients in the blood stream, and it lasts for about three to five hours. After that, you're in a post-absorptive state where nothing is digested. This doesn't stop your insulin levels in your blood from being high. At this time, your cells are starting to take up the remaining blood glucose for either storage or use. The body actively is digesting everything during these states, and your body is trying to use what you ate for energy.

The problem is that your cells can't absorb glucose from the blood stream on their own. They can only do this with insulin, and insulin is a hormone that your pancreas secrets. Insulin is meant to prompt your cells to take glucose from the bloodstream to maintain a healthy blood glucose concentration. This means that even with excess glucose in the blood, your insulin keeps your cells absorbing the glucose the excess glucose then gets converted into glycogen, which is stored in the liver.

The glycogen is your body's emergency source of energy, and when your glucose levels are too low for an extended period of time, they are used. However, glycogen stores are limited. You can only store about two thousand calories at a time, so sift there is still an excess of glucose, it's converted into glycerol and fatty acids. This means that it's being stored as fat around organs and under the skin. Therefore, insulin in your bloodstream will promote fat storage while inhibiting your ability to burn fat.

This entire process takes about ten to twelve hours after you've eaten. You won't start entering the fasting state until ten to twelve hours, but only I you don't take any better a fasted state is where your body has no glucose in the bloodstream, so your body is looking or nutrients. Therefore, it'll turn to glycogen to get the energy you need. The glycogen is then converted to glucose using glucagon, which is also a hormone that your pancreas creates. Though, the best part is at this point your body is no longer using glycogen exclusively as its energy source. It starts to use up your fat stores too, allowing you to burn fat. It becomes easier to lose weight, and that's the goal of intermittent fasting. You want to enter the fasted state by spacing your meals in a way that you're entering into this state every single day. This pushes your body to use stored fat.

The problem many people have is that they don't usually get to the fasted state. When you eat breakfast, lunch and dinner in a normal routine, you only have four to five hours in between meals, resulting in an overload of nutrition's, which keep you in the fed state. You only start to get to the fasted state when you sleep on a normal schedule, but even this is broken up when you wake up early and eat breakfast.

This has a long term effect on your body. Your body is used to burning glucose instead of fat for the energy it needs. Your insulin levels are usually always high on a normal diet, and then your cells start to become blinded to the signals, making them struggle to take up insulin. This can result in insulin resistance, which is where your body rarely ever burns fat. This means that even when your glucose is depleted your body will become hungry for more glucose instead of turning to the fat is has at its disposal. That's why intermittent fasting is the secret to weight loss success. You can eat what you want so long as you don't over indulge, but only if you're careful of when you eat. Your insulin levels fall as a result of not eating for an extended period of time. Your body is signaled to burn the fat stores it has, and this brings you weight loss in the long term.

Minimum Fasting Hours

The minimum to intermittent fasting is waiting twelve to fourteen hours between meals, but you can increase your fasting time and increase your fat burning time. Some people prefer sixteen hours with eight hours to eat for this reason. It's the best way to maximize your intermittent fasting weight loss.

Making a Motivational Choice

People usually fail a few weeks after deciding to make a dietary or fitness change because of the choices they make. They don't help themselves to stay motivated. Instead, they continue to tell themselves that they don't have the right genetics, that they don't have enough time, that it's too hard, and that they've already tried everything among other excuses. You have to make the choice to stay motivated since motivation is critical to weight los. You have to achieve clarity to achieve motivation.

Ask the Right Questions

You'll have to ask yourself the right questions if you plan to find your motivation to stick to an intermittent fasting diet.

- **Why do you want this?** You need to ask yourself why you want to lose weight with intermittent fasting. Maybe you want to impress your significant other. Maybe you want to look and feel your best in the long term. Maybe you want to feel more confident, or maybe you want to prove that you have control over your own life. No matter what the reason, this question is critical.
- **Why must you do this?** You can't think of it as an option. You have to think of this as something you must do with no exceptions. You have to determine why it must work. Write down some reasons why this has to work out for you.
- **What will happen if you don't achieve your goals?** Most of us can be easily motivated by pain, which is why we procrastinate. We associate taking on a project with pain, but eventually you complete it because the pain of not completing it seems greater than the pain of completing it. Therefore, if you find a reason why you have to do something then you'll have an easier time committing to completing it. Write down reasons or ways it'll become painful if you don't do it.

Maybe your cholesterol will continue to get worse? Maybe you're worried you won't be able to fit your favorite clothes. Just find a motivational reason why completing your goals is something that you have to do to avoid painful consequences. Even if you're just trying to avoid mental or emotional pain.

Now that you've answered these questions, you'll want to keep the answers where you can look at them. Make sure that the answers are actually written down so that you can revisit them whenever you need the extra motivation. Journaling can also be helpful, which we will cover later in the book.

Changing Your Thinking to the Long Term

People often give up if things don't line up and go the way they planned, but you have to look at this as a marathon. You're going to be able to sprint to the finish line. If you have some crazy weight loss goal that isn't realistic, you're already setting yourself up for failure. It doesn't matter who you are or what you're doing, you aren't going to lose thirty pounds in a week or less.

You could run all day and eat nothing, and you still would fall short of your goal by a mile. It's also not a sustainable strategy. You never want to pick a goal or strategy that is harmful to your health if you want to succeed. Having a healthy perspective is important to sustainable weight loss. You may not build all the muscle you hope to in a week. You may not reach every weight loss goal in a week, but just remember that at the need of the week you'll be one step closer to your goal. Every day is one day closer, and that's how you prepare yourself for a marathon and get sustainable results. While it can be great to set a goal such as I want to gain five pounds of muscle or lose ten pounds of fat, you have to realize that there's a process to it if you plan to achieve them. Instead of phrasing your goals like you want to lose ten pounds in five weeks, look at what you need to reach that goal and make that a goal. Make it a goal to stick to your feeding window each and every day for a week or to work out five times in one week. This will help you to reach your ultimate goal with a goal that is attainable.

Overcoming Excuses

Limiting your beliefs is a sure fire way to set yourself up for failure. If you allow yourself to believe the lies that come easy, such as you don't have time, or you'll never look the way you want, or you'll always stay the same, then you've already given up. Your actions follow what you believe even if you're working towards change. If you believe that you'll fail, you will fail. You enter into a self-fulfilling prophecy. Take those disempowering statements, turning them to empowering ones instead. instead of telling yourself you don't have the time, ask what you can do with the time that you do have available to you. By asking yourself an empowering question, you're regaining your power and control over your own thought process. You stop playing the victim, and it helps you to become proactive in your life. You'll be surprised with the answers that you come up with too! The answers you find will be full of perspective and positivity. Your brain is wired to answer questions, so you will come up with an answer if you ask the right questions. These questions will shake your reality. Ask yourself what lies you've told yourself that you believe, and that will give you the opportunity to replace those lies with something that gives you the power to make the changes in your life you want to.

Boosting Your Metabolism

Intermittent fasting comes for a variety of reasons, and the first one is that you create a calorie deficient, which is important to weight loss. You're also less likely to actually consume as many calories when you have predetermined window for eating. This also contributes to your calorie deficit. However, the most important reason that intermittent fasting can help you to lose weight in the long term is that boosts your metabolism. It's a common myth that skipping meals will slow your metabolic rate. This is only true with extremely long periods of fasting, but studies have proven that short periods will actually increase your metabolism. NCBI published a study that says that eleven men proved that a three day fast increased their metabolic rate by fourteen percent. It was believed to be due to the rise in norepinephrine, which is a hormone that promotes fat burning. This is a stress hormone, and it also improves attention and alertness. With more norepinephrine in your blood, more fatty acids to burn comes with it.

Waste Elimination

Another way that intermittent fasting helps to boost your metabolism is that it helps with waste elimination. With drinking and eating your body accumulates toxins, and intermittent fasting gives your body more time to eliminate those toxins and wastes because it gives you a chance to regularly clear your digestive system. This cleanses your internal organs, which in turn increases your metabolism since you won't have toxins hindering your digestion. When you do eat, your body doesn't have to use the energy to remove toxins and digest this way, allowing it to fully focus on digesting the food you eat. Your digestion is regulated because of this, allowing you to break down food and burn fat efficiently. So not only does it boosts your metabolic function but it promotes healthy bowels too.

Fat Burning Training

Your body is temporarily deprived of the sugars as well, which it's used to burning as fuel. This allows you to burn fat in the short term during your fast, resting your body during each fasting period. Your metabolism kicks up a notch and can even combat insulin resistance this way, which keeps many people from shedding the pounds that they want.

Blood Sugar Regulation

One thing that most people don't know is that hunger is caused by blood sugar levels. Your body burns fat at a steady rate with intermittent fasting, which keeps your hunger under control. This means that there is no frequent conversion and stagnation of your blood sugar levels, letting your body burn the fat it needs. This will leave you feeling sated. You won't experience this if your blood glucose levels stay high in a fed state. This will lower your risk of developing insulin resistance too. This keeps your metabolism and digestion on the right track.

Healthier Eating Habits

Most people are dependent on food, but intermittent fasting breaks this dependency. You'll gain more clarity about your eating habits and what makes you fell fuller and healthier. It helps you to understand what your body needs to run optimally. This leads to you fueling your body correctly, leaving you with a healthy metabolism and healthy energy levels. Just remember to include fiber to aid in digestion!

Slowed Aging

Intermittent fasting allows your body to rest. With less work to perform, the aging process is slowed down. By giving your body a rest, you're upping your metabolism, slowing down aging, and lowering your calorie intake. Your body will always have a faster metabolism when it's young, so aging can negatively affect just how quickly your body burns fat.

More Benefits of Intermittent Fasting

Intermittent fasting is a great way to get healthy, and it can do more than just boost your metabolism and make you lose some belly fat.

Lowers Diabetes Risk

Since intermittent fasting can help to lower your blood sugar levels and reduce insulin resistance, it helps to fight against type 2 diabetes. Intermittent fasting can reduce your blood sugar by three to six percent while staying in the healthy levels. Intermittent fasting can help protect against kidney damage as well, which is one of the more severe complications of diabetes.

Reduced Inflammation & Oxidative Stress

Oxidative stress is a step towards aging, and it can lead to chronic diseases. Free radicles react with important protein, DNA and other important molecules, damaging them. However, intermittent fasting can enhance your body's natural resistance to oxidative stress. Additional studies show that intermittent fasting can fight inflammation, which can also lead to common diseases as well.

It's Great for Your Heart!

The world's biggest killer is currently heart disease. Blood pressure, total and LDL cholesterol, inflammatory markers, blood sugar levels and blood triglycerides are risk factors associated with heart disease, and intermittent fasting can help with all of them. Just remember that you need to stick with intermittent fasting as a lifestyle if you want to reap these health benefits.

Improved Cellular Repair Processes

When you fast your cells will initiate a cellular waste removal which is called autophagy. It involves your cells metabolizes dysfunctional and broken proteins that build up inside your body over time. This can provide protection against several diseases including Alzheimer's and many forms of cancer.

It's Great for Your Brain!

Usually what's good for your body is also good or your brain. As intermittent fasting does improve metabolic features, it improves brain health. Oxidative stress, reduced inflammation and reduced blood sugar are all known to benefit brain function and nerve cells. It also increases brain derived neurotrophic factor, and a deficiency of brain derived neurotrophic factor can lead to depression and other brain problems intermittent fasting can also protect your brain against the risk of stroke.

Types of Fasting

Intermittent fasting works differently for different people, so you need to pick the fasting schedule that works best for you. Base it on your time, food portions, and the length of a fast that you want. In this chapter, we'll go over a few different types that can be used.

The 16/8 Method

We've already briefly covered this method of intermittent fasting since it is one of the most popular methods being used currently. This is best suited or the focused gym-goer who wants to lose body fat and maybe even build muscle. It's also suitable for someone who works or goes to school since it has more flexibility to plan your meals and workouts. You're eating window with this type of intermittent fast is eight to ten hours, and you're going without food for fourteen to sixteen hours. During this eating window you can at least fit two meals, but some people even eat a full three meals in this time. Just avoid meals after dinner, and try skipping breakfast to easily keep on this schedule.

So, if you have dinner at eight, then you can't eat anything until noon the next day. This is easily accomplished by skipping breakfast when you wake up. You can accomplish this even I you're a breakfast lover because you will eventually adjust. During your fast, you can drink coffee, water, and other beverages that reduce hunger so long as they don't have calories in them. This means that if you're drinking coffee or tea you need to skip the creamer and sugar until you're able to eat again.

Though, while this is an easy way to start intermittent fasting it's important to remember that you have to keep a constant feeding window time. If you don't, then your hormones can be thrown off balance, which makes it harder to stick to your diet and lose the weight you want. What you eat will depend on your work out. For example, on a day that you plant to exercise, it's okay to have more carbs than fat. Your body will use the carbs during your work out, but on other days you should have a higher at consumption. Protein should be high each day as well, but that will vary depending on your goals, age, activity level, current body fat and gender.

When you want to work out, you'll want to break your fast using fruit, vegetables and meat. However, it's okay to toss in a few extra carbs from starches such as whole grain or potatoes. Just make sure it isn't too big of a meal or you'll feel sluggish. Just make sure that you train within three hours after you eat, and then you can have a larger meal after your workout. If you want a treat, make sure it isn't too large or too high in fat. A low fat ice cream or sorbet is usually best.

On days that you aren't working out, you should aim to eat less. To do this it's best to cut down on the carbs and then eat more fiber filled vegetables instead. Make sure that your first meal is your largest, and your meals should get smaller as the days go on. Forty percent of your calories should come from proteins, and fatty meats such as ground beef and salmon are okay.

For your last meal during the day, make sure that you include a protein fish or meat is fine so long as you have fiber and vegetables with it. This will help keep you full during your fast because you have a good supply of amino acids. A fast won't work if you consuming loads of junk food right before it. You'll feel hungry and your body won't have the nutrients it needs to start shedding those pounds. Whole and unprocessed foods are better versus liquid or processed foods.

The best part of this type of intermittent fasting is that you don't have to plan your meals at certain types. During your feeding window you can eat whenever you want and what you want within moderation so long as you try to keep a balanced meal. It also works for hormonal control. Another great advantage of this method is that you are eating the same way each and every day, so you don't have to worry about adapting your body to an erratic schedule. However, this method does require that you eat a certain way right before and right after you work out if you want this intermittent fasting method to work for you.

Alternate Day Fasting Method

This type of fasting is better suited for serious dieters that have their weight loss goals denied. It's also called the up and down day diet, which means you fast every other day. There are different variations of this type of fasting, and it's not recommended for the average person just wanting to lose a few pounds or keep their weight under control. One popular method of the alternate day fast is instead of having no food one day you limit yourself to 500 calories. Another version of this is where you eat a fifth of what you would on a normal day for your fasting day. So for example, if you eat 2,000 calories a day, then on your fasting day you'd limit yourself to only 400 calories.

If you're a beginner, this wouldn't be the best intermittent fasting method to start with. Though, this method is based on cutting back calories, which is a sure fire weight loss plan. Though, it can be difficult to work out on the days you aren't eating. So, you'd need to work with less strenuous exercises. Exercise is important for this type of intermittent fasting, and many people fall prey to binging during normal days. If you do want to try this method, try to plan your meals ahead of time so you know exactly what you're eating.

The 5:2 Method

This intermittent fasting method is best for people who have less time in their schedule, so they'd normally have a hard time following a strict meal plan or eating regime. With this type of diet you eat normally for five days, and for the remaining two days you limit your calorie intake. Usually people eat only 500 to 600 calories on those two days, and it was a method that was popularized by Michael Mosley, a British doctor. It's known as the Fast diet, and women are recommended to consume 500 calories during their two day fast and men are recommended to consuming 600 calories.

With this type of intermittent fasting, your days to not have to be consecutive. Therefore, you can take Monday off and then Thursday off and have the weekend free, or you can choose the two days that are best for you. It's actually less effective to choose two days back to back. For this method to work, you need to have at least one non-fasting day between them where you eat normally.

For the days that you do fast, you will want to choose two to three small meals to count for your calorie intake so that you aren't getting all of your calories at once. Just keep in mind that eating normally doesn't mean you're able to eat anything you want. If you eat tons of junk food, you're more than likely to gain a few pounds than lose them. There aren't any rules on what you eat on the fast day, but there are generally two meal patterns some people will eat three small meals including a breakfast, lunch and dinner so that they don't feel as hungry during the day.

Other people prefer to eat two meals that are slightly bigger. With only two meals a day, most people prefer to skip breakfast. Since your calorie budget is limited, it's important to plan your meals accordingly. Try to stick to high fiber foods that are low in calories so that you stay full, and pick out protein that is nutrient dense to make sure that you get all the nutrients you need. Soups are a good example, but so is cauliflower rice, berries, eggs, lean meat, grilled fish, and even black coffee. This type of intermittent fasting is effective at weight loss and reducing insulin levels. It can improve insulin sensitivity. Sadly, if you make the wrong food choices, then you can actually gain weight using this routine.

The 4:3 Method

This method functions almost exactly like the 5:2 method, except that you have an extra day with extra calorie restrictions so that you can meet your weight loss goals faster. However, if you can't stick to the 5:2 method, then you won't be able to stick to the 4:3 method. Work with the 5:2 method first, and then add in the extra day as you get used to it for the best results.

The Eat Stop Eat Method

This is good for already healthy eaters that just want to lose a little more weight. This is an intermittent fasting method where you have a twenty-four hour fast once or even twice a week. You'd not eat from one dinner to the next which provides a twenty-four hour fast. This will reduce your calorie intake without actually limiting what you're able to eat. With this method you need to practice regular workouts to reach your goals faster and keep your body healthy and running smoothly.

Just eat normally during your feeding period. You'll need to keep yourself occupied during your fast. Just make sure that you drink enough liquids and get regular sleep to make it easier. During your fasting period you shouldn't take in anything that has calories. This type of fast is easier for people who don't want to regularly limit themselves, and you don't have to dive into it all at once.

Some people start with an eight hour fast once or twice a week and start to slowly work the time up. One week it'll be eight hours, the next time it'll be ten, and so on until you reach a full twenty-four hour fast. Another great part of this type of intermittent fasting is that there isn't any forbidden food and you don't have to count calories either. This makes it easier to follow for most people. Just use moderation.

The downside to this type of intermittent fasting is that it can be challenging to go a full day without food. This is why it's advised to start small and prolong your fast each week. You might experience headaches, fatigue, crankiness and dizziness during your fast, but the effects usually diminish over time. It can also be tempting to binge once your fast is over, but with self-control and meal planning, this can be managed.

The Warrior Method

This is a rule based approach to intermittent fasting that you need to be committed to if you want it to work for you. It's a popular approach that involves eating raw vegetables and fruit during the day and a warrior sized meal at night. So, you can feast at night within a four hour window if you fast the rest of the day. Fasting in this case isn't actually avoiding food, which makes it easier to stick to. What you eat and when you eat is key to making this method work.

The food choices that you eat with this intermittent fasting is similar to the paleo diet. You need to concentrate on food that is unprocessed and whole. They should be foods that look like they do in nature. This lets you fuel your body with the nutrients that you need. The fasting phrase of this method is that for twenty hours you eat only a few servings of vegetables, fresh juice and just a little bit of protein. This maximizes the fight or flight response, which stimulates fat burning, promoting an energy boost and alertness. The hour window is your overeating phrase, and it's meant to maximize the ability of your parasympathetic nervous system to asset your body in recuperation, promoting relaxation. This lets your body use the nutrients that it's taken to repair itself and grow.

Eating during the day can assist your body in producing the hormones you need too, as well as burning the fat you want to lose. The best part of this type of intermittent fasting is that it has clear guidelines on what you can eat, but that can also be restrictive to some people. By being able to eat small snacks during the day, your energy levels are increased too, allowing you to work out a little easier. Sadly, this can also interfere with social gatherings since a strict meal plan for twenty hours can often interfere with social gatherings.

Skipping Meals Spontaneously

With intermittent fasting, it's about making the choices that fit you. A defined fasting plan isn't always necessary. You can always skip meals spontaneously and still lose weight. You can always skip meals when it's convenient, such as when you don't have time to cook or eat. It's a myth that people have to eat every few hours. You won't start losing muscle and you won't enter starvation mode. Your body is equipped to handle extended courses of famine, so skipping a few meals from time to time can be the push your body needs to start burning fat. If you aren't hungry during a meal time, you don't need to force yourself to eat. Just skip it and wait until your next meal. Don't give into the temptation of junk food!

About Liquid Fasting

There are liquid fasts as well, but you'll want to think of these as a temporary diet and not a lifestyle. In this chapter we'll explore water fasting, liquid protein fasting and juice fasting.

Water Fasting

This is a quick way to detox your system, and it has a strong impact on getting your body back on track. Though, it is one of the most difficult fasts to take on. You'll need to ready yourself a few days prior to your water fast or you won't be able to stick to it. Though, it can be a challenge emotionally as well. Some people prefer to have professional supervision when doing a water fast, but if it's less than three days it is safe for the average person. A normal water fast has a zero calorie admission. This means you only drink water, and you don't add anything to it. With this type of fast, you aren't adding any nourishment to the body. Nourishment acts as a roadblock to a complete resting state, so you won't be able to completely cleanse or detox your body.

It's one of the most extreme ways to detoxify your body. The first thing you need to realize is that water fasting isn't suitable to be constant, frequent, and it isn't for everyone. Some people see their skin clear up, pain lesson, and other small issues clear up almost immediately with a water fast. During a water fast, it's recommended that you consume two quarts of water every day. You'll want to either use a pure water or at least a distilled water. Distilled water is bad for regular consumption, but adding it into your water fast can be a huge help to removing toxins. After two days your body will go into ketosis.

You will feel hungriest on the first day, but that hunger will significantly decrease over time. If you want to do a water fast, then you'll want to do it when you don't have to drive or go to work. The point where people can safely work in ketosis varies from person to person, so it's best not to do anything that puts you or others in danger. You'll want to consider being supervised if you're trying to use a water fast to help with serious conditions or you've never tried a twenty-four hour water fast before. If you are overweight, you will also want to have supervision during a water fast.

Liquid Protein Fast

It is easier for your bodies to eliminate and work through liquid than it is for your body to work at breaking down whole food. That's why a liquid protein fast is a great way to lose weight without losing muscle. Most people will opt for protein shakes when dealing with this type of fast, and it'll keep you feeling full longer. Other people prefer to cut down their calories while using a liquid protein fast as well so that they lose weight. Once again, it's best to only do this fast for about three days before switching back to a normal diet. It is not a type of fast that you should do too often.

Juice Fast

Someone on a juice fast is going to consume nothing but juice, and they'll need a juicer too. You don't want to drink store bought juice and expect it to work out for you. Most juices are loaded with sugar, but you'll find there are some juice fast diet plans out there where you can buy your healthy juice in advance. Just do your research or make your own!

With a juice fast, you'll drink only juice in place of solid food for a few days. The amount of juice is between one to two liters a day, and in between your "meals", you may also drink plenty of water, herbal teas and some juice fasts let you drink vegetable soups. However, it's important to realize that most intermittent fasts do not include a juice fast since they aren't meant to be made into a regular diet or lifestyle. However, some people prefer to kick off their intermittent fasting diet with a juice fast to completely detoxify their body.

When Not to Liquid Fast

You shouldn't do any sort of liquid fasting if you're hypo-glycemic, hyper-glycemic, nursing, pregnant, have just undergone surgery, have dealt with an eating disorder or are daily prescription medication. If you have a liver or kidney disease, have low blood pressure, a terminal disease, are anemic, or any other chronic condition, then you shouldn't use a liquid fast either. If you are unsure if you should use a liquid fast, then consult with your doctor before starting any type of liquid fast.

A Lesson in Food

If you want to use intermittent fasting to meet your weight loss and health goals, you have to take a look at the food that you're putting in your body during your feeding periods. That's why it's important that you learn a little more about food. Food has changed over the years. The food was simple back in history, but now there are corporate giants that are using steroids into their meet and spraying their vegetables with pesticides. Worse yet, you have junk food on the shelves that have little to no nutritional value while giving you nothing but empty calories and blood sugar spikes.

The end goal with intermittent fasting is to prevent inflammation, shed the pounds, and boost your energy levels in the process. Intermittent fasting allows you to reach these goals with moderate exercise and healthy eating. To make your feeding window count, you need to know what food is composed of so you can make an educated decision on what to eat and what to avoid. The first thing you need to realize is that food is made of macronutrients. They consist of protein, carbohydrates, also known as carbs, and fat. Each one has a role in your body, so let's take a look at what that role is.

Protein

Protein is important in building muscle mass, and it's necessary for cell regeneration, skin elasticity, oxygen transport and immune function. It's compromised of amino acids, which are smaller molecules. Amino acids function as the building blocks of protein, and protein is the building block of muscle. Any animal or animal by product has protein in it, including beef, chicken, turkey, fish, eggs, bison and dairy products. If the food you're eating once was alive or came from something that was alive, then it has protein in it. Meat is a complete protein, so they have a large spectrum of amino acids. This isn't the case with plant based proteins, which will be covered later in the chapter.

Carbs

Carbohydrates, also known as carbs, and it's a common myth that weight gain is caused by carbs. Carbs are important in the body, but you don't want an excess of carbs. Carbs are your main energy source, and if you don't use them instantly then they're toted in the muscle and in the liver. This forms glycogen which causes fat. There are various vitamins and minerals in carbs, and it's where you get your fiber a cup of barley contains ten grams of fiber, seven grams of protein, selenium, phosphorous, manganese, and even copper. These minerals are considered to be trace minerals, and they're proper for bodily systems including brain function.

Barley is considered a whole grain, and carbs are in whole grains and whole-grain derivatives. Beans, potatoes, fruits and a handful of vegetables is also a source of carbs. What you want to avoid is simple carbs, such as potato chips, crackers, cakes, bread, cookies and other refined and highly processed foods. Simple carbs can also be found in sweetened teas, fruit juices and other beverages such as soda. You'll even find simple carbs in alcohol.

You should also know that there are some carbs that are high in protein, but that doesn't mean that they're complete proteins. For protein to be complete it has to have essential amino acids in it. Animal products are complete proteins, but most protein containing carbs aren't. In fact, soy beans area one of the few carbs that have complete proteins in it. If you're vegan, you can get complete proteins rom plant-based sources such as whole grains, certain vegetables and beans. It's a common misconception that you need to include these items in the safe meal to get what you need. As long you eat a few incomplete proteins in your diet throughout a twenty-four hour span of time, you'll be okay.

Fat

Fat was demonized in the early to mid-80s because many people believed it's what caused weight gain, but this isn't true. It also isn't the leading contributor to heart disease. Still, the general public believes that fat is bad for you. You actually need to avoid low-fat and no-fat foods because they're loaded with sugar, which actually does cause weight gain. Sugar is carbs, and carbs have calories. The carb content of low-fat and no-fat food is extremely high. Low-fat and no-fat products give you a false sense of security to eat what you want.

Fat actually is a macronutrient that is needed in your body. Fat is essential for hormone production. Hormones circulate through your body to allow your body to go about its daily routine. Hormones contribute to your ability to lift weights, concentrate, reproduce, and so much more. Without hormones functioning properly, your body won't work properly mentally or physically. Fat is essential for brain function, inflammation reduction, energy and skin health too. Physical fat on your body is meant to protect your organs and insulate you from the cold too, but if you have too much it'll cause chronic health conditions. Though, just like carbs you'll find that there are good fat and bad fat. Unadulterated fats such as olives, coconut oil, red palm oil, nuts, seeds, cold water fish, and olive oil are good fats. Healthy fats are great for your body. Bad fats are fats that have become carcinogenic or have been highly refined.

Hydrogenation takes place when hydrogen atoms are added to an oil such as soybean oil during manufacturing. The oil breaks down at high heat which is when it becomes hydrogenated. A product that has been hydrogenated has a longer shelf life, and hydrogenated or partially hydrogenated oils are saturated fat. The actual fat doesn't harm the body, but the combination of simple carbs and saturated fat is detrimental to your health and weight loss goals. The rule of thumb is never combine saturated fat with simple carbs, but that doesn't mean you have to avoid either of them completely. Just make sure you aren't eating them together.

Some Exceptions

Before you decide to cut out saturated fat and cholesterol completely, you need to realize they're the main force behind testosterone and human growth hormone. If you want to gain muscle, then you can't cut it out completely. Just approach eating them with caution and moderation. Coconut oil and red palm oi are saturated fats, but they're actually healthy. Just make sure you aren't getting the refined or processed kinds. If you want to build muscle, then get a little saturated fat in your diet each and every day, but never go overboard. One to two tablespoons is best, so a good quality egg can help your diet a lot. Pork rinds are actually a great thing to sneak into your diet since they are high in protein and fat, but make sure you get ones that are free of hormones and antibiotics. Just get enough of these types of fat and cholesterol to spark hormone activity, but don't go overboard.

Keeping Balance

Macronutrients play a vital role in your body, and without them you would have a hard time surviving and staying healthy. Though, people who follow low-carb or no-carb diets usually will try to convince you otherwise. It all comes back to balance, so make sure that you remember to eat everything in moderation. Just be aware of what you eat and drink, but the best part about intermittent fasting is that you're able to follow any diet you want and still benefit from it. You can even get away without eating super healthy or on a health strict diet and still obtain some of the benefits from intermittent fasting, including some weight loss.

Protocols to Follow

There are some protocols you need to follow for both mental performance and nutritional performance. The mental performance protocol is up to you, but it will make reaching your goal easier.

Mental Protocol

In this book, we've already talked about how your mental performance is essential to meeting all of your health and weight loss goals. With intermittent fasting, you should be able to reach an intense level of focus. Think about it in the terms of lunch time. If everyone at lunch goes to blow their budget and meal plan on lunch, they'll have massive insulin spikes which will also cause a massive crash later. While they struggle to regain their focus, your focus is already there because you didn't receive that massive insulin spike. Intermittent fasting can change the way you focus on your work and projects so that you increase your personal performance.

Take in a little caffeine in the morning to help out. If you're worried you're going to get addicted, then drink something like green tea. It'll wake you up, suppress your appetite and help you to focus first thing in the morning. What most people don't know is that caffeine also is proven to boost your memory, increase your reaction time, and even increase logical reasoning. It can also help to reduce chronic inflammation. The next step is to drink a second cup of something that's low in caffeine when you start to feel hungry. You can skip this step later on, but when you're just getting used to intermittent fasting, it's recommended for your mental health.

It'll help you to push your fast forward so that you don't break it as quickly. Just remember that caffeine in the evening may affect your sleep, so skip this step if you're already experiencing issues sleeping. After this, make sure that your first meal is always after two in the afternoon. Even if you just started. This will keep you focused on your task during the day because your body isn't focusing on digesting food.

If you absolutely have to break your fast before two, then eat something like an apple which only has about one hundred calories. This will help to restore your glycogen and keep you feeling full without wasting your focus. If you're just getting started with intermittent fasting, use this mental protocol before you actually settle into an intermittent fasting method. It'll prepare you to commit to whatever method you choose.

Nutrition Protocol

Depending on what your goal is will depend on what nutrition protocol you'll need to follow.

For Extreme Weight Loss

Only use this protocol if you're looking to lose a lot of weight in a short amount of time. The first thing you'll need to do is learn to calculate your calorie budget. Now, let's put that "quick" weight loss into perspective. Losing one to two pounds a week is considered quick if you are between ten to fifteen percent body fat. If your body fat is already higher than this, you'll often see more substantial results. So, take your goal weight and then multiply it by ten.

This is a good way to calculate your calorie budget for both men and women. If you're a man that weights two hundred pounds but you want to weigh only one hundred and eighty pounds, then you'll want to eat 1,800 calories which is one hundred and eight times ten. This will allow you to lose the weight you want. Now, eating this little with intermittent fasting is easier since you don't have to try to split that calorie amount by four to six meals. Now, let's break this math down so that you can understand it a little easier. An average male that weighs 180 has a TDEE of 2,500-2,800. So, if they ate around 2,650, then they'd maintain their weight. However, cutting it down by 850 calories to make it 2,650, they have a deficit of 850 calories. Not eating 850 calories each day over a week will make a 5,950 calorie deficit. Nearly 6,000 calories! This will equal almost two pounds of body fat lost in one week since a pound of body fat has 3,500 calories in it.

If you're using this type of nutrition protocol, you'll want to follow it for eight weeks at a time before re-evaluating your weight loss goals. If you can commit for two full months, you can then either choose to continue with tis protocol by redefining your goal, or recalculate it so that you are maintaining your weight. Another reason you should only follow this nutrition protocol is because your body will get used to it. Your metabolism will down-regulate, which means the weight loss you experience initially will begin to stall because it has reached homeostasis. When you rebuild your metabolism, then you'll be able to enter into another weight loss protocol method.

For Building Lean Bulk

You'll want to use this nutrition protocol if you're already happy with your fat levels and just want to build up some lean muscle. The traditional bulking method is ineffective for most people since it causes people to pick up a lot of weight which is mainly fat, and then they don't usually successfully lose that excess fat later. With this bulking method, you're less likely to pack on a few extra pounds of fat instead of muscle. You get to cut out the ineffective bulk and cut cycles.

To start this, you're going to have to calculate your maintenance calories. You can usually find a TDEE calculator on the internet, which is important to helping you get the right number. Just take it with a grain of salt since they'll likely overestimate the amount of calories you need, which can lead to some fat gain. If you don't want to use an online TDEE calculator, then take your body weight and then multiply it by fourteen if you gain weight easily or if you don't gain weight easily multiply it by sixteen. If you feel you're in the middle, then times your body weight by fifteen instead. For women, it's recommended that you stick with fourteen since women traditionally gain weight easier than men.

Once again, let's take a 180 pound man as an example who gains weight quickly. They'd then take their weight and time sit by fourteen to get 2,520 calories. That would be the amount of calories they need to maintain their weight. Now, for lean bulk you only want to add 180 calories more than your maintenance calories. This will ensure that your body gets the calories it needs to build up lean muscle without packing on fat. Just keep in mind that you aren't going to build muscle if you aren't exercising. Instead, that 180 calories will turn into fat. Now, remember that about 2,500 calories are in a pound of muscle.

You'll only pack on about a half a pound of muscle per week with good circumstances and still build muscle in a healthy way. This means that you need about 1,250 calories to make that half a pound. Divide that by seven days and its 179 calories a day, which is where the 180 calories comes from. However, if you're following this type of nutrition protocol and see that your waist measurement is going up, which you'll want to measure every day, then reduce it by fifty to one hundred calories a day.

Building muscle will depend on your body. Keep in mind that when you're packing on lean muscle, your weight will go up. You just don't want your waist measurement to go up. If it does go up by a little, that means you're just packing on your muscle in the abdomen region, but if it goes up too much then you're packing on fat. You'll need to combine it with a muscle building protocol or this to work.

For Muscle Gain & Slow Fat Loss

You'll want to use this protocol when you want to gain muscle but still lose some fat. Just remember that you'll both gain your muscle and lose the fat slowly. You won't see drastic results quickly. This will help you to build muscle and lose fat each week, even if it's just a small amount. On training day you'll want to eat a calorie surplus, and on days that you're resting you'll need to take a calorie deficit to use this. It's also referred to as recompesition.

Start by calculating your calorie budget by calculating your maintenance calories. On rest days a 180 pound man would need to eat 400 calories under their maintenance calories. On training days, they'd need to eat about 300 calories over their maintenance. In the week, the calorie surplus needs to equal about zero. Just don't expect results too quickly, but you'll be sculpting your body to what you want

For Metabolic Rate Increase

You'll want to use this nutritional protocol if you're eating very little but still having a hard time losing weight. It's also meant to help increase your metabolic rate. You'll also want to use this if your goal is to enter an active fat loss period later on in your goals. Remember that long terms goals are better than short term goals so long as you realize that you have to work on the short term too.

Your body's goal is to stay alive, but it can make fat loss hard for many people. When your body realizes that it's starving it shows down functions in such as slowing down your metabolic rate. This is so that you can stay alive for longer even if you're starving. Your body has a hard time telling the different between when you're enduring famine and when you're trying to lose weight. If you're eating next to nothing but still having a problem losing weight, you'd need to go into a reverse dieting phrase to actually correct your metabolism. Otherwise, you won't make any weight loss progress.

This is a tool that you can use to up-regulate your metabolism, and then once your metabolism has returned to normal you'll be able to enter a weight loss phase. However, you should keep in mind that reverse dieting requires a high level of commitment because it's extremely specific. If you aren't careful, you'll actually gain weight with this method. However, if you do it correctly you can have incredible results and get your weight loss back on track. Your results are dependent on your natural body composition as well as how close you follow your protocol.

Imagine that if you eat 2,000 calories to maintain weight and then you cut it back to 1,500 calories you expect massive fat loss. You may lose this initially, which usually shows up as two pounds per week if you aren't severely overweight. Eventually though, your body adjusts to the small amount of calories so that you hit a plateau. During this phase you stop losing the weight you want. Most people would continue to cut their calories at this point, but after a few months you could be eating as little as 1,000 calories.

Your body may readjust yet again, which means you won't lose weight despite eating such a small amount. This is where most people start to ail and lack the results they want. During this phase you might go out to eat a dinner that's 2,000 calories with friend, and then the extra 1,000 calories is then stored as at, so you're going to actually gain weight with just one slip up. Your body is just trying to keep you alive because it believes that you're experiencing an extended period of famine. It only takes one night out to have your weight go out when you're at this stage, which would make most people start to freak out when they hop on the scale and get the bad news. They'd then cut back their calories again, but at this point that isn't helping. You have a yo-yo diet effect where you eat very little and still don't lose weight because your body has achieved homeostasis. Then you can binge eat or eat just a little too much and gain fat. This will make many people freak out and go back to eating very little until they once again eat homeostasis until they eat too much again and it all happens all over again. Reverse dieting is the only effective way to break out of this habit.

For the first day, determine the current calories you're eating using a food calculator. For the point of argument, we're going to use the example of 1,500 calories. On the second day, you're going to want to determine what your target macronutrients are. Your protein consumption should be one gram per pound of body weight. So if you weigh 150 pounds, then you will want 150 grams of protein. Then you'll want to subtract the protein calories from your current budget. So with 150 grams of protein multiplied by four calories per gram then that's going to be 600 calories from protein. Now out of 1,500 calories with 600 of it being from protein it means that you have 900 calories remaining. Then you'll split these 900 calories between carbs and fat.

Sixty percent of it should go to carbs and forty percent should go to fat. So that's 540 calories from carbs and 360 from fat. Now, let's calculate how many grams of carbs and fat that equals. With four calories per gram, you'll want divide your number of carb calories by four. This will make 135 grams of carbs. For 360 calories from fat divided by nine calories a gram, you'll get 40 grams of fat. Now you know your macro targets. Eating this would make your weight stay the same overall. Though, you may gain or lose a bit depending on how long it takes your metabolism to balance out.

The next step is to determine how quickly you'll increase your carbs and fat weekly. If you increase it too quickly you'll pick up more fat, but this is good if you want to focus on eating normally more than you're worried about gaining weight. This speeds up the process a bit. If you want to start weight training, you can be more aggressive about adding on calories. Weight lifting will slow down some fat gain that's associated with reverse dieting. If you binge eat or break your diet often, then you'll want to go aggressively bring up your calories quickly. Though it'll lead to weight gain initially it will negate the yo-yo diet effect.

The next step is to decide on three days of the week that you weight yourself or take your stomach measurements. For some people, it's best to do both. This will help measure your progress. Now, don't let that make you feel bad. The scale is just a tool that measures your weight, and you have to remember that it doesn't measure your worth. Don't let the number on your scale scare you, and it's normal for your weight to go up and down by up to two pounds a day.

The next step is to decide on the speed you want to reverse diet. If you want an aggressive approach then up your carbs and fat by six to ten percent a week. You won't need to adjust your protein since you've already optimized it. If you want to go slowly, then only up your fats and carbs by two to five percent a week. If you've added five percent of the calories back without picking up weight, then your body is adapting well, which is the best results you can hope for.

You can then become more aggressive with your reverse dieting. However, if you have increased it by two to five percent and are still picking up weight then you shouldn't adjust anything. Most people freak out and drop their calories back to where they started, but this will only increase the yo-yo effect, which isn't what you want. Your metabolism will eventually level out, and you'll just need to put up with the weight gain until it does. When it does level out, you can increase your calories by two to three percentage until you get your metabolism back to normal.

After you're done reverse dieting, which may take a few weeks to a few months, then you can enter a fat loss program. However, some people do choose to continue to reverse diet until they reach an upper threshold to determine their metabolic ability. The higher you can take your metabolic ability the easier it'll be for you to diet and build muscle in the future, but you run the risk of gaining more weight in the meantime.

Other people choose to maintain the weight they've gain by stopping the addition of calories and instead continue to use a calorie maintenance formula. Though, most people will want to use a fat loss program at this point. To start this you need to lower your calories, and then you can use an aggressive approach by using the extreme weight loss protocol. If you aren't worried about losing weight too quickly you can try a more controlled approach which would require lowering your daily calories by about 250 to 500 calories. By lowering your calories that little you can lose up to a pound a week. However, if your weight loss stalls, you'll need to lower your calories again.

Intermittent Fasting FAQ

In this chapter we'll go over some of the more commonly asked questions about intermittent fasting and their answer so that you can start your new diet with confidence.

Is intermittent fasting for everyone?

Yes, anyone can use intermittent fasting so long as they don't already have existing health concerns that restrict their diet. You can use intermittent fasting with allergies, but not if you already suffer from heart disease, gastrointestinal disease, and other serious medical conditions. If you do, then you'll want to talk to your doctor before trying intermittent fasting.

Is changing my diet necessary to benefit from it?

While changing your diet to healthier foods will increase your weight loss results when using an intermittent fasting method, you do not need to in order to benefit from intermittent fasting.

Will I lose my muscle by using intermittent fasting?

No, you won't lose your muscle by fasting. Actually, fasting in this manner is a great way to maintain your muscle while still losing weight. Sadly, that means the scale may not be the best way to measure your health goals. Remember that you want to cut down on your body fat, not just your overall weight.

Is this good for my life expectancy?

Actually, intermittent fasting will help you to live longer since you're consuming few calories. You're still getting all the calories and nutrients you need to keep your body healthy and young, so you'll be healthier overall. Your health often determines your lie expectantly.

Is one method better than the other?

No, one method of intermittent fasting isn't better than the other. It all depends on the type of goals you have and how your daily schedule looks. Just pick the method that works best for you, and if one doesn't work out well, then try something else. Remember that skipping meals is an option too!

Isn't fasting bad for your blood sugar?

In the long run, fasting is great for your blood sugar since it resets your body. It's a myth that low blood sugar is a common problem. Healthy people can maintain a healthy blood sugar level in a variety of situations, including fasting. While your blood sugar will lower during a fast, if you're healthy, it should not reach hypoglycemic levels.

Is exercising necessary during fasting days?

While exercising during your fast is recommended, it is not necessary in order to reach your weight loss goals. Since fasting often limits your calorie intake, weight loss will come naturally, but many people hit a plateau. By exercising, you're more likely to improve your overall health and get over the weight loss plateau faster.

What if I've stopped losing weight but I'm eating very little?

This means your metabolism has adjusted to the amount of calories you're taking in. This can happen even if you're eating well below your maintenance calories. In this case, you need to lower your calories while still in a healthy zone. If this continues, then see the reverse diet protocol to bring your metabolism back up.

Should I weigh myself every week?

While you can weight yourself every week if your goal is to mainly lose weight, it isn't needed to measure your intermittent fasting success. It's better for some people to measure every two weeks or to measure their waistline instead of their weight on the scale. No matter what you do, make sure that you aren't measuring your weight more than once a week. Keep in mind that it is normal for your weight to fluctuate some each day, so measuring every day will only discourage you.

Doesn't breakfast start your metabolism?

This is a common myth. There is no actual need to start your metabolism. Even without food in your stomach, your body will use the fat in your body as fuel, so you don't need to eat breakfast.

Are headaches normal when fasting?

Not everyone will have headaches when fasting, but a lot of people do. Women are especially susceptible to headaches during fasting. It's a common misconception that this is due to dehydration. Actually, it's commonly believed that it's withdrawal symptoms. It's similar to the headaches that people experience when they quit coffee cold turkey. For example, you're cutting down carbs, so you may have headaches from that. Your first couple of fasts will be the most difficult. Just treat your headaches like you normally would, but make sure to stay hydrated to help alleviate symptoms even if it isn't due to dehydration. Dehydration can still make it worse.

What if I've already damaged my metabolism?

It's actually unlikely that you've actually damaged your metabolism. The human body is incredibly adaptable. This means your body can survive on little to no calories. Metabolic damage hardly ever occurs, so it's likely that instead you've experienced metabolic adaption. Just take a deep breath, and then try the reverse dieting section to get your metabolism back up to normal.

Can you drink alcohol when fasting?

While you can, it isn't recommended. No matter what type of intermittent fasting method you practice, you do want to limit your calories. Alcohol is usually full of calories because it's mixed with something. Beer and wine do have calories, and they are empty calories. They don't provide you with any vitamins or nutrients. While liquor is often calorie free, it can lead to dehydration and make side effects from a fast feel worse, such as headaches, hunger pangs, or even dizziness. It's best to stick with black coffee, unsweetened tea or water during your fasting days. If you want to drink alcohol during you non-fasting days, just make sure that you're mindful of the calorie intake.

Is it normal to feel cold when fasting?

Fasting will increase blood flow to body fat, which can cause you to feel cold. It's completely normal, and there's nothing to worry about. When you're fasting more blood travels to your body fat causing vasoconstriction to occur in your fingertips and toes to compensate. However, if any numbness occurs, you should talk to your doctor.

What if I don't see result after two weeks?

If you don't see any results in two weeks, then you'll want to ask yourself if you've really stuck to your intermittent fasting method. If you aren't, then you need to re-commit to it. If you did stick to it but still don't see results, you may need to reset your metabolism by reverse dieting or choose an intermittent fasting method that works better for you. Remember to accurately calculate the amount of calories you need to lose weight.

Intermittent Fasting Precautions

Intermittent fasting can be incredibly beneficial to your health, but it does have some drawbacks, and it's isn't for everyone. It can be beneficial to some people, but others shouldn't use it. So take these precautions before starting an intermittent fasting lifestyle.

Check Your Blood Sugar Levels

Before you consider intermittent fasting you need to check on your blood sugar. If you suffer from diabetes or low blood sugar, eating regularly is vital in making sure that you remain healthy. With these conditions, going long periods of time without eating can lead to drastically low blood sugar levels even though it wouldn't cause issues in most people. Dangerous complications can result from someone fasting with diabetes such as shakiness, heart palpitations and fatigue. It's important that you consult your doctor before starting intermittent fasting as a diet or a lifestyle to see if it's right or you.

Look at Your Eating History

It's important to avoid intermittent fasting if you have ever suffered from an eating disorder. Regardless of it it was when you were a teen or an adult, not eating for a long period can trigger old symptoms and unhealthy eating habits. It can push you back into a negative headspace which could risk your health.

Look at Your Age

Children and teenagers shouldn't use an intermittent fasting method. Intermittent fasting is meant to be handled by healthy adults. There is no need for children or teenagers to go on large fasts, especially when they're still growing and need the extra nutrition. Children and teenagers should only watch what you eat. A healthy diet is good for anyone.

Don't Do It When Ill

When you are sick, your body needs the extra nutrition to heal and get better. Therefore, you should avoid intermittent fasting when you're sick or you'll slow down your healing process. Remember that nutrients are essential to immune function.

It May Not Be For Most Women

There is a lot of factors for women to consider before they start using the intermittent fasting method. You should avoid intermittent fasting when pregnant or lactating. By limiting you're eating window, then you're limiting the amount of nutrients you're providing for your unborn child, and it'll reflect in your breastmilk too. Instead of fasting, just try to eat a balanced diet instead. Sadly, for women long term intermittent fasting can also lead to hormonal issues, which could cause an issue for weight loss as well. It can also interfere with regulating menstruation cycles, menopause, puberty, hair growth and even skin complexion. Some women should only use intermittent fasting for a few days or a few weeks instead of using it as a lifestyle. It's suggested that you keep a journal if you want to use intermittent fasting as a lifestyle. If you start to have issues that don't diminish after a few days or are severe, then you'll need to stop the intermittent fasting diet or consult your doctor.

Avoid If You Have Gallbladder Issues

If you already have gallbladder problems, then you need to avoid intermittent fasting since it can increase the risks associated with gallbladder issues. If you have a history of gallstone disease, intermittent fasting would be unwise.

Look at Your Thyroid History

Intermittent fasting can alter hormones, which includes hormones that regulate your thyroid. If you have a history of thyroid issues or if thyroid issues run in your family, then you may want to avoid intermittent fasting as well, especially long term.

If You Really Love the Gym

While you can exercise while using the intermittent fasting diet, it can be much more difficult. If you don't want to take a break from the gym or change the way you exercise, then intermittent fasting may not be the best diet or lifestyle for you.

Side Effects & Solutions

Like any change to your daily routine, you'll need to get used to intermittent fasting. Of course, like any diet or lifestyle change, it may come with side effects that you can avoid, especially during the transition period. In this chapter we'll go over some of the most common intermittent fasting side effects and how to avoid them.

Losing Muscle

While intermittent fasting usually burns fat and not muscle, you can lose muscle if you aren't using intermittent fasting properly. In general, intermittent fasting should not burn muscle mass. If you're on a diet with a lot of carbs, you're at a higher risk of increased gluconeogenesis with periods of fasting, which will result in some muscle being burned. What you need to do is rest, cut back on the carbs, and increase your sodium intake slightly. Training while you fast can also help you to keep your muscle mass by causing a greater anabolic response once you eat again, allowing you to build your muscle back up as long as you're getting enough calories and proteins.

Your Mood Drops

While intermittent fasting should not affect your mental clarity, it can cause aggravation and irritability as well as snappiness, avoidance, moodiness, exhaustion and lethargy. A warm cup of coffee can often give you the energy you need to liven you up as the caffeine increases fat oxidation and releases adrenaline. This should remove the mental fog. Other than that, you just need to give your body time to adjust to your new fasting lifestyle. Try to eat something before or during social interactions, so schedule your fast around your schedule or vice versa to improve your mood when around others.

Digestive Issues

Diarrhea and constipation can be an issue when you start fasting for the first time. This is your body striking back against your new dietary changes, but it will become less of an issue after you get used to the new routine. Just remember that it's temporary. If you feel constipated, then try drinking more water, adding more fiber to your meals, consuming more potassium, and adding electrolytes to your diet. If you have diarrhea, after breaking your fast, you may want to try charcoal tablets or herbal teas.

Macronutrient Deficiencies

I you don't eat for days on end, your body isn't getting the essential nutrients it needs such as vitamin B12, potassium, magnesium, omega-3s and more, but this is why you shouldn't fast for long periods of time. Just make sure that you are only fasting for a restricted time window. Prioritize nutrient dense foods such as unprocessed meats, fish, healthy fats, eggs and vegetables to makes sure your body doesn't run low on these essential macronutrients to keep your body running smoothly.

Adrenal Fatigue

You're asking for trouble if you pair intermittent fasting with negative habits, strenuous workouts each and every day, stress, and overexertion. This will cause adrenal fatigue. Usually this is a side effect because you are using intermittent fasting with an already unhealthy and negative lifestyle. Just make sure you don't fast too frequently or for too long. If you're having this issue, try a 16:8 method.

Mistakes to Watch Out For

The best way to make intermittent fasting work for you is to avoid the most common pitfalls. In this chapter we'll go over the most common mistakes people make with intermittent fasting and how to avoid them.

Being too Full After Eating

When you're used to eating several meals a day, it's easy to consume enough without worrying about being too full. However, if you're working with a small feeding window, you have to eat a few big meals. This can leave you feeling uncomfortably full after breaking your fast, and it can cause constipation. You'll also find that your quality of sleep can suffer at night if you eat a big meal before bed. Most of the time, you'll find your hungry once you are able to break your fast, so eating a food immediately after breaking it is normal. However, just pace your meals throughout your feeding window. Don't let yourself get to this point. Two to three small meals is easier than trying to consume one or two big meals during your feeding period.

Being Obsessed with Your Feeding Window

Your life should not revolve around food. If you obsess over eating, you're going to overeat. You can overeat even on healthy food. Don't count don your hours until you're able to eat again. It'll lead to an obsession that will harm your diet plans in the future, making it impossible to turn intermittent fasting into a lifestyle that you can commit to. Becoming obsessed with food during your feeding window will lead to forced weight loss, but you'd gain the weight back in the future.

Becoming Reliant on Caffeine

While coffee can help you to get through the hunger and control your appetite, you can't become overly reliant on coffee to stay energized and expect intermittent fating to work for you in the long term. Drinking coffee on a regular basis can lead to an addiction, which can cause stress, anxiety and poor sleeping habits. It can even cause weight gain to return.

Giving in to Food Cravings

Hunger is going to be a challenge no matter who you are when you start intermittent fasting, and food cravings come with it. During your feeding window, you are able to eat, but sticking to healthy food is important. Often, your cravings will be or salt and sugar which can push back your weight loss goals. Just realize that so long as you make sure that you get proper nutrition these cravings should diminish over time.

Over Exercising During Your Fast

While exercising can help you to get through intermittent fasting, you shouldn't over exercise. Athletic performance will naturally diminish when fasting, so long intervals of exercise can cause you to eel achy, more fatigued, and extra hungry before your fasting period is over. So, if you do exercise make it light exercise or short bursts that don't over exhaust you.

Dealing Poorly with Heartburn

Many people experience heartburn when practicing intermittent fasting for the first time, but it usually will rectify itself over time. For many people they'll see improvement within three weeks, but for other people it can take up to six weeks to see results. If your heartburn doesn't go away after six weeks, you'll want to consult your doctor. Heartburn is normal as your body gets used to a new way of eating. With heartburn your body is releasing acid at certain times because it's used to needing that acid at that time. Just treat the heartburn as you normally would, and try to stick it out. Giving up because of heartburn is a sure fire way to fail to reach your weight loss goals

Dealing with Headaches Poorly

Headaches are a common occurrence during intermittent fasting, especially for women. This will also go away, but dehydration is going to make it worse. If you deal poorly with headaches, then it can easily put a dent in your intermittent fasting plans. Try herbal teas to relieve headaches and hydrate at the same time!

Becoming Reliant on Naps

While it's easy to get through your fast by napping or most of it, over sleeping will cause headaches and other problems. It can also stress you out, so it's important to only take a nap when you really need it. If you become reliant on taking a nap to get through your fast, you won't burn the calories you need to in order to reach your health goals. Napping will also slow down your metabolism since your body doesn't need to burn as many calories when you're sleeping.

Expecting Too Much Too Quickly

If you expect to lose weight too quickly, then you're going to think that the intermittent fasting diet won't work for you. If you set your goals too high, you're giving yourself too much room for failure. Work on small changes that you can get through before moving on to the next change. For example, work on cutting one meal out a day before trying to cut out two or before trying to cut down your meal size. Work on six hours of fasting before working on eight and so on so that you increase your likelihood of succeeding.

Thinking that Longer is Better

Intermittent fasting is good for you, but only in moderation fasting for twenty-four hours can be healthy, but you shouldn't push yourself to fast for forty-eight or seventy-two. Fasting benefits start to dwindle after about twenty hours, so you don't really want to fast for more than twenty-four. More isn't always better in this case, so don't try to extend your fasting hours too far.

A Gradual Transition

Now that you know intermittent fasting can help you with your weight loss goals, you just need to know how to get started. It can be hard to transition to just not eating for an extended period of time without any crankiness, dizziness or hunger. You need to slowly incorporate intermittent fasting as a part of your life. In this chapter, we'll explore a few ways that you can get used to intermittent fasting so that it's easier to utilize as a weight loss tool.

Start by Setting a Goal

Before you start, try to determine what you want to achieve before you start fasting. With a goal in mind, it's easier to reach those goals. It gives you mental fortitude to withstand the fasting period without giving into temptation. Some goals you can set are reducing the time you spend eating, which will prevent excess weight gain. It can also help prevent liver damage. If your aim is to reduce the time you're eating, then the warrior diet may be the best intermittent fasting method.

If you want to extend your lifetime expectancy by reducing your overall fat and help with your cholesterol levels, then any method of intermittent fasting can help. Intermittent fasting helps to lower blood pressure levels, reduce fat, reduce cholesterol, and reduce blood sugar, which can help you to extend your lifespan. However, it only works if you accompany our intermittent fasting with a low carb diet and moderate exercise. Intermittent fasting works best when you avoid processed and refined foods.

If your goal is simply relieve inflammation in your body, then intermittent fasting can help with that too. A restricted eating time increases bile acid production, which will help improve adipose tissue homeostasis, which alleviates inflammation. In this case, any method works, but the 16:8 method works best. If you're trying to reduce inflammation, you'll also want to cut refined flour, vegetable oils and dairy to help reach this goal.

Actually Getting Started

So, now the question is how do you actually start. Once you decide on the type of intermittent fasting you want, then you need start by planning your first few weeks. Make sure that you get out a calendar, and make sure you actually know when you want to fast, especially if you aren't using a standard method. You just need to make sure that you're committed, have a plan, and you are willing to deal with the transition period. If you are used to eating every three to five hours, then you're going to feel hungry. If you're jumping in to a restrictive diet, it's going to be hard to stick to. You just need to remember to do it gradually. If you go all in, then you're just inviting disaster. If you've never fasted before, it'll be harder to get started.

Work On Your Sleep

When you're sleeping, it's easier to fast. It's easier to go without food when you don't notice the time passing. It's natural to look forward to when you eat next. You just have to realize you can't base your life on when you can eat next or what you eat next. Fasting should be seen as a normal part of our daily routine, and if you feel too overwhelmed, then take a nap to help pass the time. This can't be done each and every time, but it's a great way to get started and catch up on some extra sleep at the same time. Eat when it comes to easting time, but make sure to eat healthy. Remember that it's harder to lose weight when you aren't getting proper sleep. Sleep helps you to reset your body.

Allow for a Detox

It's important to reduce the irritating symptoms of toxicity if you want to use intermittent fasting properly. A natural detox is one of the best ways to ease yourself into a fast. Just start by altering your diet to kick out processed foods such as granola bars, protein bars, soda, sugar and processed meat. Once your system is clear, it's easier to start fasting since your insulin levels won't be fluctuating nearly as badly.

Choose Your Last Meal Carefully

Your last meal can make or break how easy it is for you to start and stick to your fast. If you're eating something that has nothing but empty calories, you're going to derail your fast before it even begins. Don't get fast food. Cook a whole meal that most of your time fasting is spent digesting the food that you just ate. Avoid large amounts of sugar and carbs for your last meal since they'll only make you hungry early on. A sugar rush is always followed by a sugar crash and hunger pants.

Fighting Off Hunger

You're bound to feel hungry when you're fasting at one point or another. That doesn't mean that there isn't anything you can do to keep hunger pangs from setting in to badly. In this chapter we'll explore how to manage your hunger to stick to your fast.

Drink Water!

Staying hydrated makes fasting easier to get through. Thirst can easily be confused for hunger, so when you're feeling hungry, try drinking a glass of water. Just make sure that you don't chug it or you can upset your stomach! This is your best tool against hunger.

Drink Tea or Coffee

Other than water, tea and coffee can help you to stave off hunger too. Just remember that you shouldn't use any sweetener. Caffeine and other stimulants work as an appetite suppressant. Caffeine will stimulate the hormone cholecystokinin (CCK), which your body releases after it's eaten. It'll give you a feeling of calm, and it'll help you to feel full even without eating a meal. It will also hydrate your body to boost your energy level and provide you with antioxidants. Don't wait for the hunger to kick in full force, when you start to feel hungry then start preparing a cup to help you get through it.

Start Exercising

You'll want to start exercising in short and intense bursts. Doing this during a fasting period will keep your mind from focusing on the hunger you're experiencing. Sprinting or lifting weights are great examples of an intense but short exercise that you can do to stave off hunger. It's also a great way to boost your muscles and blast away fat. The best part is that this type of exercise is known to suppress your appetite.

Different types of exercise will affect your body in different ways. Aerobics, for example, will suppress ghrelin, which is a hormone that increases your appetite. It also increases the production of peptide YY which will decrease your appetite. So, it's best to do twenty minutes of this exercise when you're about to finish your fast so that you don't overeat when you eat your first meal. Over eating would be counterproductive.

Try Meditation

If you stay relaxed, you'll get through your fast a lot easier. Meditation is a great way to solidify your self-control and get you to relax. Anxiety and stress will trigger you to want to eat, and that's where meditation can work miracles. As you get better at mediation, it becomes easier to control your hunger. It'll help you to avoid temptation in the meantime and gives you something to concentrate on.

Do Some Chores

Keeping busy is important to avoiding hunger. If you aren't working during your fast, it can be harder. That's why it's important to start looking for something else. Either chores or a hobby can do the trick when staving off hunger. Cleaning or gardening will keep you focused on a task, and it's especially important when you're just getting used to intermittent fasting. You can even take this opportunity to start your own garden, as home grown food is a great way to make sure that you stay on track with your diet goals. For the same reason, if you have something that you've been putting off. Even if you're just been putting off deleting things in your email, then this would be the time to do it. Focus on something other than your hunger.

Try Walking

If you aren't quite up to exercising and can't think of anything else to do to keep your mind off of hunger, then try to take a walk. A brisk walk will help increase your fat burning, and it'll take up some of your time. Combine your fast with a regular walking routine, and you'll actually lose more weight. Take your dog for a walk, go to buy groceries, or just try a scenic walk around your neighborhood.

Munch a Little

This should be a last resort, but if you absolutely can't control your hunger then you'll need a controlled fast. A controlled fast is just where you eat foods that have a low glycemic index. This means that the food have the least impact on your blood sugar levels. Unprocessed fruits and vegetables are what you'll want to stick with. Do not cook them, and you'll still want to keep them to small servings.

Intermittent Fasting & Building Muscle

You already know that muscles are the engines your body uses to propel itself forward to do what it needs to be done. There is a direct correlation between how you treat your muscles and how you grow your muscles. When you go to lift an object your brain sends a signal to your limbs. For example, if you pick up a cup of coffee your bicep contracts and triceps relaxes, which lets you pick up object.

If you are trying to pick up something larger, then a larger signal is sent to your brain. This means that more motor neurons are fired. When you place your muscles under more stress than they're used to, then microscopic damage occurs. Cytokines are then released by the damaged cells. Cytokines are inflammatory molecules which active your immune system to repair the damage and start muscle growth. The greater the damage the more that will need to be released to repair the damage.

Your muscles are already adapted to everyday tasks so when you do everyday tasks you aren't putting any stress on your muscles. Hypertrophy is the stress that's needed to build muscles. To expose your muscles to hypertrophy you have to expose them to a high volume. Of course, if you stop exposing your muscles to stress or tension, then they'll start to shrink as well which is known as muscle atrophy. This is one reason that protein is so important. Remember that protein is the building block for your muscles!

Terms to Know

Here are a few terms you'll need to understand if you want to build up your muscles.

- **Volume:** There can be a difference between volumes in your training. A body builder will train a high volume than a power lifter, which is why they gain muscle easier. Volume is sets multiplied by reps and then multiplied by weight.

- **Strength Training:** Strength training is another word for weight lifting, and it's one of the most effective ways to build muscle.
- **Intensity:** Think about it in terms of one rep maximum. It's a unit of measurements that indicated the amount of weight you're able to lift in a full repetition. Intensity is then defined by this value.
- **Failure:** You want to push your muscles to failure when training, which is when you are unable to complete a rep. this means that you're failing to complete the full range of motion required for the exercise. The set is complete when you reach failure. This means you've sufficiently exhausted your muscles which will help you to build muscle up later.

Using Progressive Overload

This is an important principle if you want to build muscle. You need to increase the weight, repetition and sets of your exercise, and if done right you'll get continuously stronger. It will continue to put your muscles under new stress causing microscopic tearing that allows you to repair and build your muscles up. You'll need to use a progressive model to achieve progressive overload. This is a strategy that determines when you should add more volume to your workouts.

Use a weight that allows you to fail in a given rep range. You'll want to continue to push yourself each and every week if you can exceed your suggested rep range, then increase the weight for a set by five pounds until you are unable to increase the weight .then you can add an additional set instead. so if you are benching 185 and you want to do between four to six reps. In the first week you may be able to achieve failure at four reps. At week two add another rep and you should achieve failure at five reps. By week four you should achieve failure at seven reps which surpasses the four to six rep range. At week five you'll want to start over by trying to do our reps again but by adding five pounds to bench 190.

Pairing it with Intermittent Fasting

While you can build your muscle and lose weight on intermittent fasting, it's going to be hard to do it at the same time when using intermittent fasting. Instead, you'll want to concentrate on one at a given time, and then increase your muscle later on. If you choose to lose fat first, then just try to keep your muscle up while you lose the weight so that it doesn't go through atrophy, which will make building your muscle later a little easier. Though, if you've just started weight training it is much easier to build muscle and lose weight simultaneously.

More Tips & Tricks

Even now that you know how to pick an intermittent fasting diet that will work for you and how to stave off hunger, it can still be hard to get used to this type of diet. That's what this chapter is meant to help with. Here are a few more tips and tricks that you can use to get through your first few times fasting and stick to a diet that will help you to reach your goals.

Think Differently

You shouldn't think of fasting as denying yourself food. Instead, think of it as taking a break from eating. Just take it as a break from having to worry about when you'll eat and what you'll eat, which can be stressful, especially if you have a busy schedule. During your fast, food is one less think that you need to worry about, and that can help you to stick to your fast with less issues.

Fill Your Schedule

This may seem counterproductive, but filling your schedule can actually help you to avoid temptation! If you keep busy, then you won't be sitting there on the couch where your chances of snacking are much higher than if you keep busy. So if you're just starting to commit to fasting, then over commit your schedule for a while so that you don't have to worry about snacking or sitting around with hunger pangs. This would be a great time to start volunteering or help out a friend!

Go to the Gym

If you pair consistent exercise with intermittent fasting you're going to get the best results. Just remember that light exercise is all that you need. You don't need to do more than basic training, and depending on your intermittent fasting method, you might not even need to do fully body training.

Give it Three Weeks

You have to at least try intermittent fasting or three weeks before you give up. If you can commit for three weeks and follow the method you choose, then it gives you enough time to get used to it as well as start to see results. Your body needs time to adapt, so just check the progress of your goal after at least three weeks, but most people see the best results in four to six weeks because they've gotten used to the routine and it has become a regular part of their lives.

Don't Talk about It

Intermittent fasting may have become popular, but there are still a large number of skeptics. There are even more uneducated people that don't understand the perks of fasting. Some people think that you're trying to starve yourself or that you've gone crazy, and skepticism when you're trying to commit to something makes it harder to commit. People's words can sting and invite negativity, which will make your symptoms seem even worse. It can also make you more impatient for results when your body is trying to reset so that it can finally start shedding those pounds!

Utilize Your Protein

It's important to pack protein in the meals that you do eat. . Protein will help you to build muscle. It's our nature to eat meat, so you shouldn't try to stay away from it. An intermittent fasting diet should not be paired with a vegan diet or it'll be harder to stay full.

Get Rid of the Junk

When you're using an intermittent fasting method, you already know that the junk food isn't your friend. You should use this as an opportunity to kick junk food from your life once and for all, and that starts with your pantry. Get rid of the junk food from your home before you start your fast, or the temptation will be that much worse. It's already hard to stick to a healthy diet with how easy it is to get access to fast food, but with it out of your house, it becomes a little easier. You'll want to change your buying habits to reflect you commitment too. Get rid of the alcohol, soda, chips, and even granola bars. Clean them from your cabinet and instead replace it with healthy snacks such as fresh vegetable packs, fresh fruit, and low calorie sweets I you need something for a treat.

Intermittent Fasting & Sleep

Some people have a hard time sleeping when they start fasting, but it does get easier. Proper sleep is essential in maintaining your health, which is why in this chapter we'll take a look at some tips and tricks to help you sleep.

Help Your Liver Out

When fasting, it's critical that your liver gets the assistance it needs to help with the increased work load. It may have a hard time processing the toxins that have been released in your blood stream. You can help your liver by drinking plenty of water to help eliminate those toxins, but make sure you don't drink too much right before bed. It's best to drink up until seven. Some fresh lemon juice in your water can help you to wake up in the morning as well as waking up your lemon the lemon promotes your liver and digestive system to start working. A tablespoon of apple cider vinegar in your water can help as well because it has the same alkalizing and detoxifying effects. It also helps to replenish your gut bacteria, adding in your body's elimination and digestion.

There are some herbal supplements that you can use as well including Dandelion Root and Milk Thistle, but never add a supplement into your daily routine without talking to your doctor first. Milk thistle and dandelion root helps your liver with elimination, and you can usually find these at a local food store the best part is that it's completely natural, so you aren't adding any more chemicals to your body.

Make Sure You're Eliminating Properly

If you aren't eliminating properly by having regular bowel movements, then it can affect your sleep. It'll be harder or you to excrete the toxins from your body if you're having constipation issues. It can cause general feelings of unwellness and trouble sleeping. To help with this, you'll want to add more fiber to your diet. Add in food that supports your liver, aids in digestion, and aids in elimination. Just make sure that you pair these foods with plenty of water.

Dark leafy green vegetables such as silver beet, spinach and kale are great sources of fiber and they're full of nutrients too. Fermented foods are also great at replenishing your gut bacteria. Kim Chi and Sauerkraut are great options too. You may even want to try coconut water kefir. Wholefood supplements are good to help as well too if you can't adjust your diet enough to help!

Lay Off the Caffeine

Caffeine adds stress to your liver, and it can stimulate a stress hormone in your body. If your liver is busy trying to detoxify your body, then adding caffeine to the workload is bad for your body. If you're having issues sleeping while using the intermittent fasting diet, then you need to get rid of caffeine. At the very least, you need to cut back on it. Don't drink caffeine late in the day, and think about switching to a drink that has less caffeine than coffee. Green tea is a great substitute.

Managing Your Calories

You know that to lose weight you need to reduce your calories, and intermittent fasting will help just make sure that you manage your calories appropriately to make weight loss easy. Intermittent fasting will help you or reduce your calorie intake with easy, making weight loss simple. By restricting the amount of time you have to consume food, your calorie intake is naturally restricted as well.

A Look at Calories

You burn calories with everything you do. Your calories are your energy budget, and you have to achieve a healthy balance. In a technical sense a calorie is the energy it takes to raise a kilogram of water by a single degree Celsius. Everything you eat contains calories, and they're stored in the food's chemical bonds. The calories are then released through digestion. You use calories in three areas. Ten percent of calories are used in digestion. Twenty percent of your calories are burned through physical activity, and seventy percent of your calories are burned by your body's basic tissues and organs. The seventy percent is known as the Basil Metabolic Rate. The BMR will tell you the amount of calories you need to stay alive even if you eat nothing and did nothing all day. Add digestion and activity to the mix, and then you get what's called your Total Daily Energy Expenditure (TDEE). The average guides is 2,000 calories for women and 2,500 for men. This is based on the average physical activity, weight, age, and muscle mass.

The average guidelines for BMR for women is 1,400 and for men it's 1,750. It doesn't mean that every guy can eat 2,500 calories. Think about it this way. If someone was running a marathon, they'd burn about 2,600 calories. So, if the average guy that had a BMR of 1,750, then to run a marathon they'd need 4,350 calories to maintain their weight for that day because they'd burn 2,600 calories. Though, there are factors that alter your BMR.

This includes gut bacteria, enzyme levels, intestine length, and thyroid functionality. These vary depending on the person. If you're worried about one of these variables, then you'll need to talk to your doctor.

Maintaining Your Weight

However, if you're not trying to lose weight but instead just maintain your weight, then you need to manipulate your calories accordingly. Remember that weight largely depends on an energy balance to the ratio of calories that you're consuming and expensing. If you're not using an intermittent fasting method that has you count your calories, then just try to pay attention to how many you're eating.

Though, if you're more active then you will need to add more calories. If you're less active then you might want to consider 1,200 to 1,500 calories instead. You can always adjust your calorie intake based on what you're doing that day as well. On a day that you're going to be more active, a few hundred more calories won't hurt nearly as bad since you'll be expending those too.

The basic weight loss formula is to eat less than you burn, but to gain weight you need to eat more than you burn. If you follow a weight loss formula, you'll be losing fat. Fat contains approximately 3,500 calories fore very pound. That means you need to burn 3,500 calories over your maintained calories to lose a pound of fat. The inverse is also true through. If you take in 3,500 more calories than you need, then you'll gain a pound of fat. Now, for muscles you have about 2,500 calories in every pound of muscle. With an intense strength based workout plan, you'll likely pack on a half a pound of muscle each week. This means you need to give your body the calories it needs to gain muscle. If you're trying to gain muscle, then just eat 1,250 calories over your maintenance calories to gain the muscle, which is about 180 calories per day and pair it with your workout.

Online Calculators & Other Tips

Consider using an online calorie calculator if your recipes or food don't tell you what you're consuming. If not, you might want to look at the back of the nutrition labels when you're eating prepared or packaged foods. Even many fast food chains are telling you the exact calories you're consuming when you buy a sandwich or some other type of food from their establishment. Just remember that not all calories are created equally. The lesson in food chapter should have taught you that balance is key, but even when eating poor calorie choices that aren't nutrient dense, you can still maintain or lose weight with the intermittent fasting diet. Just try to restrict your empty calorie consumption.

Intermittent Fasting & Social Gatherings

It can be hard on any diet to stick to it and still have a social life, but intermittent fasting can be particularly difficult since you might want to go out during your fasting period. In this chapter we'll explore some things you can do to make it a little easier.

Only Go Out When You Can

If you're just getting started, it'll be best to avoid social gatherings until you get in the swing of things. It can be hard to avoid temptation if you are just starting intermittent fasting. Give yourself a week before attending any big social events, especially parties where a lot of food is involved. If you do need to go out before you're ready, try to make it a short rip out. Excuse yourself if you feel like you might give into temptation!

You should never be ashamed or hesitant about your diet choices. Of course, it can also be helpful to not let people know that you've started intermittent fasting at these events. People have a habit of trying to talk you out of it or various reasons. For some people it's because they don't understand what it is, others think that you're harming your body, but usually people are just ill informed. Still, if you're trying to avoid temptation, it won't help if you have someone trying to get you to eat something when you're on your fast!

Take a Water Bottle

If you're going to be around food, take a water bottle with you. Remember that hydration is your friend, so take something with you to keep you hydrated. If your stomach is full of water, then you're going to feel a little less hungry. Even if you smell delicious food. If you're having a real hard time, then pack some green tea or unsweetened coffee instead of water, especially if you're going out in the morning.

Eat Before You Go

This won't work if you have to go during your fasting window and you're doing a full fast. Of course, if you're able to eat before you go, then it's going to help to do so. If you have calorie restriction fast, then you'll want to make sure that you choose this option. It'll let you eat something you know stays within your calorie budget while still providing you with the nutrition that you need. It can alleviate a lot of the stress that you get from going out if you know exactly what you're doing, and if you're a little fuller, it's easier to avoid temptation.

Eat at the Event

This may seem counterproductive, but if you have the option then take it! This works great if you're doing a modified fast that isn't strict on calorie counting. I the social gathering is in the evening, then just try to go throughout the day without food so that you can get your calories when you do go out. Then you don't have to avoid temptation at all.

Take a Break

It is also possible to take a break from time to time. Just like you take a break or when you're ill, you need to take a moment away from your intermittent fasting from time to time. Even if you've chosen intermittent fasting as a lifestyle. If you don't allow your break from time to time, then you're going to take a break when you shouldn't. So, if you want to take a break for your friend's special day or for the holidays, then do so. Don't try to make it up later either or you'll end up going overboard. Instead, you'll want to just go back to your normal routine. Just remember that your body may have side effects as it tries to get used to intermittent fasting again if you broke your fast too much, consumed too many calories, or did it for too long.

Keeping a Fasting Journal

If you plan to use intermittent fasting to reach any type of goal or use it in the long term, then you will want to create a journal to track your progress. It can also give you the mental push that you need in order to stick to your fast even when you want to give up.

Make it Portable

When you're keeping a journal to help with intermittent fasting, you'll want to be able to take it with you. After all, you don't want something bulky. You also don't want to try to remember everything when you get home. Just make sure that you keep a small pen with you and your journal so that you can jot down how you feel, what your progress is, and what you've eaten or drank throughout the day. You'll want to write down any symptoms you're experiencing, what you drank, what you ate, and if you've seen anything positive that is helping you with your fast.

Start with Your Goals

Outline your goals in the first page of your journal, and leave enough room to track your progress for a few weeks. If you backslide from your goal, then you'll know to adjust something in your intermittent fasting diet so that you can reach them easier the next week. If you are reaching your goals with ease, then you know that you're on the right track to reaching your goals. When you do reach your goals, then write another page with another goal, even if you're just looking to maintain the weight.

Write Frequently

This is the main reason you want your journal to be portable! You can't expect to remember everything that happens during the day, especially if you're dealing with intermittent fasting symptoms. Therefore you'll want to make a habit of when to pull out your journal. Never be ashamed to write in your journal in front of people, but at the very least keep your journal in your car so that you can write in it before you go home after an event.

Keep it Positive

Writing down positivity can help you to stay positive during your fast when you start lacking motivation. When you go back through your journal it can also be important to be able to re-read those positive thoughts. If you didn't get a headache after your fasting period, write it down. If you lost a pound since last week, write it down. If you weren't as hungry after drinking another cup of water, then write it down.

Go Back Through Your Journal

Every few days you'll want to go back through your journal to determine if you're getting sick because of something that you're eating or drinking. Some people have food allergies that are so mild that they don't notice them when they're eating or drinking a lot, especially if it doesn't appear as a serious allergy or intolerance. You may find that coffee upsets your stomach by causing too much acid, which means your body is intolerant to coffee. If you notice this trend, then you'd be able to modify your fast to avoid coffee while replacing it with something else that can help you such as black tea or green tea.

You may also notice that certain foods upset your stomach, and you'd want to avoid these. Headaches can come with certain food intolerances too. Use your journal as a way to modify your behavior and fast later on. If you find that a certain feeding window doesn't work for you, then try to adjust your feeding window to a better schedule so that it's easier to stick to your intermittent fasting lifestyle or diet.

A Little about Exercise

While exercise isn't necessary to lose weight with intermittent fasting, it is recommended since it'll help to speed everything along. It's also a critical part of a healthy lifestyle. Cardio is recommended when intermittent fasting. There are a few different types of cardio that you can use for fat loss, and you can choose an intensity level based on your health and weight loss goals.

Walking

Walking burns roughly 300-400 calories an hour. It's great for beginners, and it's good for people who have previously been injured. It has a low intensity, and it's suggested you do it three to six times a week. For each walking session try to make it twenty to forty-five minutes at a time.

Running

Running burns about 600 calories an hour because it requires a higher intensity. Though, it's considered a high impact exercise which can hurt your joints in the long run. So you'll need to be careful. If you want to use running as your cardio, it's recommended three to six times a week. You should run for at least twenty to thirty minutes at a time.

Cycling

This is a low impact cardio that also burns about 600 calories an hour. Once again you'll want to do this three to six times a week for a twenty to thirty minute session.

Rowing

This is a higher intensity exercise that burns about 840 calories an hour. It's suggested you do this for thirty to forty-five minutes at a time three to six times a week.

Jumping Rope

This is another high impact activity, but it can give you a great workout when done correctly. It burns about 1,000 calories an hour too! It's suggested you use it three to six times a week, but you should only use it for fifteen to forty-five minutes a session.

Yoga

Yoga is a low impact activity that will help you to increase your muscle strength, muscle tone and flexibility. It's recommended that you do it for an hour, and depending on the positions it can burn from 200-600 calories an hour.

Conclusion

Now you know everything you need to in order to start intermittent fasting to reach your weight loss and health goals. Intermittent fasting is best when used as a lifestyle rather than a diet, but it can be used either way depending on your own health goals. However, just keep in mind that there is more than one approach to intermittent fasting, and you'll need to pick the type of intermittent fasting that works for you and pair it with other healthy lifestyle choices to reach the best results! With the right intermittent fasting method for you, all of your health and weight loss goals are within reach.

www.ingramcontent.com/pod-product-compliance
Lightning Source LLC
Chambersburg PA
CBHW070030260726
48658CB00002B/576